Contents outline

Transform Your Body and Mind in a Minutes

"If you're stuck in a routine office job or find yourself going through the same motions as a housewife day after day, it can be easy to feel trapped and uninspired. But the truth is, you have the power to change your life and transform your daily routine into something that energizes and empowers you. By incorporating morning exercise into your routine, you can boost your physical and mental well-being, increase your energy levels, and start your day with a sense of purpose and accomplishment. It may be challenging at first, but with dedication and persistence, you can create a morning exercise routine that transforms your life and unlocks your full potential."

Preparation

This is me whose writing, telling you about real experience, we are all in somehow prefer sticking to usual routine and avoiding any extra effort. After all, it's familiar and comfortable, right?

This is what exactly was in my mind before I created a new healthier routine, I wasn't look for good shaped body, I was looking for healthier life style, believe me bad old habits deserve to be fought, I know we all have enough on our plates with bills, relationships, bosses, commutes, and chasing our dreams, too much pressure so waking up in the morning and start exercising doesn't seem to be the good option in the middle of all that but common let's face it many studies have shown that a lack of exercise can have negative effects on an individual's health. A study published in the Lancet medical journal found that physical inactivity is responsible for approximately 6% of all global deaths. another study published in the American Journal of Preventive Medicine found that prolonged sitting time is associated with increased mortality, regardless of physical activity levels. Physical activity has also been shown to have positive effects on mental health, with regular exercise being linked to lower rates of depression and anxiety. So get up buddy and don't let your bad habits beat you down, don't ever let your mind play you and tell you that you don't have extra 30 minutes or less a day, 5 times a week, actually you do, it is just matter of mind, time is there and had never been changed, every day is 24 hours; was and will continue to be.

Believe it or not life is a battle field and it needs warriors to go through, warriors in life mean a healthy person physically and mentally, it is way much better to fight in this life with better health and clear mind.

Since Corona lockdown I started and I'm doing this now because I need it, it is not exercising anymore, it is a life style I have chosen and hopefully I will continue.

I choose to write this to transfer the happiness that I found; it will be selfishness if I keep it all to myself.

The Benefits of Morning Exercise

There are many reasons why people choose to exercise in the morning, and the benefits are numerous. One of the most significant benefits of morning exercise is that it helps you jump-start your day with a burst of energy. By engaging in physical activity early in the morning, you increase blood flow and oxygen to the brain, which can help you feel more alert and focused throughout the day.

Moreover, morning exercise can help to regulate your sleep cycle. Exercise has been shown to improve sleep quality, which can help you fall asleep more easily at night and wake up refreshed in the morning. Research has also shown that morning exercise can improve your metabolism and help you burn more calories throughout the day, leading to weight loss and improved overall health.

Furthermore, morning exercise can improve your mood and reduce stress levels. Exercise releases endorphins, which are feel-good chemicals that can boost your mood and reduce feelings of anxiety and depression. By starting your day with a positive and energized mindset, you can set the tone for the rest of your day and tackle challenges with greater ease.

When it comes to the best time to exercise, many experts recommend exercising in the morning. This is because our cortisol levels are highest in the morning, which can help to increase our energy levels and reduce the risk of injury. Additionally, exercising in the morning can help to regulate our circadian rhythms, making it easier to fall asleep at night.

Overall, the benefits of morning exercise are numerous and well-documented. By incorporating regular exercise into your morning routine, you can improve your physical and mental health, increase your energy levels, and experience a greater sense of well-being.

Examples of Exercises

There are many different types of exercises that men and women can incorporate into their morning exercise routine. Here are a few examples:

- Cycling or running is a great cardiovascular exercise, cycling was my choice at the beginning and still.
- Jumping rope is a great form of cardiovascular exercise that can improve your fitness level, coordination, and endurance, also it is a great alternative if weather conditions don't help for running or cycling.
- Push-ups: This exercise works your chest, arms, and core muscles.
- Pull-ups: This exercise works your back, shoulders, and arms.
- Squats or lunges: This exercise works your lower body, including your glutes, quads, and hamstrings.
- Stomach exercises can improve core strength, posture, athletic performance, digestion, reduce the risk of injury, and enhance appearance.
- Plank: This exercise works your core muscles and can help to improve your posture.
- Yoga: This exercise can help to improve your flexibility, balance, and
- overall mental and physical health.
- Burpees are a full-body exercise that involves a combination of squatting, jumping, and push-ups, and can help to improve cardiovascular endurance, strength, and overall fitness.

Cycling in the morning is a great cardiovascular exercise that offers numerous benefits for the body and mind. Like running, cycling can help to improve cardiovascular health, boost metabolism, and aid in weight loss or management. Cycling is also a low-impact exercise; However, the amount of time spent cycling can vary depending on factors such as fitness level and goals. Additionally, incorporating interval training or hill work can help to increase intensity and challenge the body. Cycling in the morning can also be a great way to enjoy fresh air, improve mood, and increase mental clarity throughout the day.

Running in the morning has many benefits for both the body and the mind. Firstly, it can help to boost metabolism and kickstart the body's natural fat-burning process, which can aid in weight loss and weight management. Running in the morning can also help to increase energy levels and mental clarity throughout the day, as well as promote better sleep at night. Additionally, running can help to reduce stress and anxiety levels, which can have a positive impact on overall mood and mental health.

Jumping rope is a popular cardiovascular exercise that requires coordination, endurance, and agility. The basic technique involves holding the handles of a jump rope and swinging it over the head, jumping over the rope as it passes under the feet. To start, beginners can practice by jumping with both feet together, gradually progressing to more advanced techniques such as alternate foot jumps, double-unders, and criss-crosses. Proper form is crucial to avoid injury and maximize the benefits of the exercise. This includes keeping the elbows close to the body, using the wrists to turn the rope, landing softly on the balls of the feet, and maintaining an upright posture with the core engaged. With consistent practice and proper technique, jumping rope can improve cardiovascular health, coordination, and overall fitness.

Push-ups are a classic exercise that can be performed in a variety of ways, depending on your fitness level. Start with a basic push-up by placing your hands on the ground shoulder-width apart and lowering your body until your chest nearly touches the ground. For a more advanced variation, try a diamond push-up by placing your hands close together in a diamond shape.

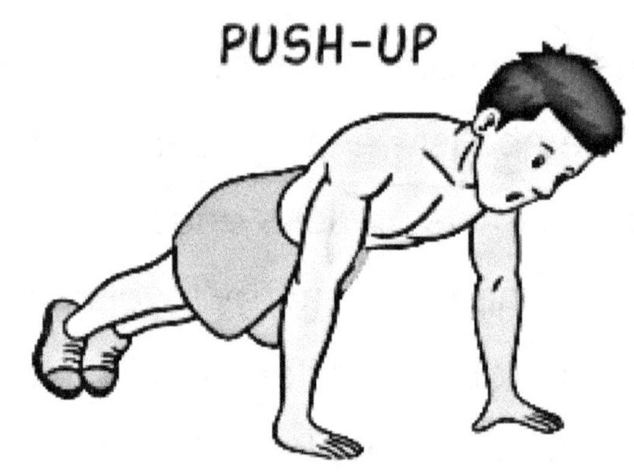

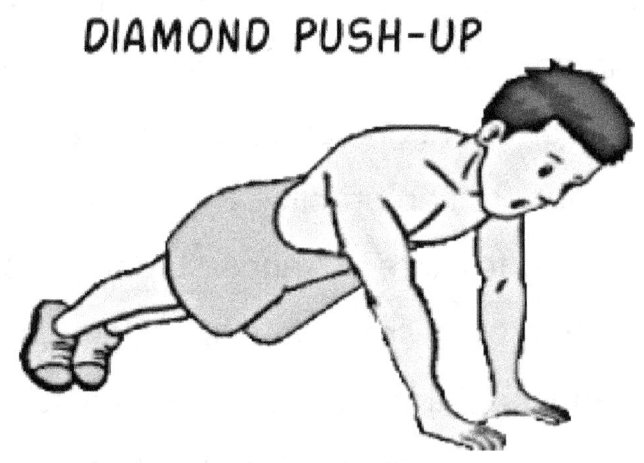

Pull-ups are a challenging exercise that can build strength in your back, shoulders, and arms. To perform a pull-up, start by hanging from a pull-up bar with your palms facing away from you. Pull your body up until your chin is above the bar, then slowly lower yourself back down. If you're new to pull-ups, you can start by using an assisted pull-up machine or resistance bands to make the exercise easier.

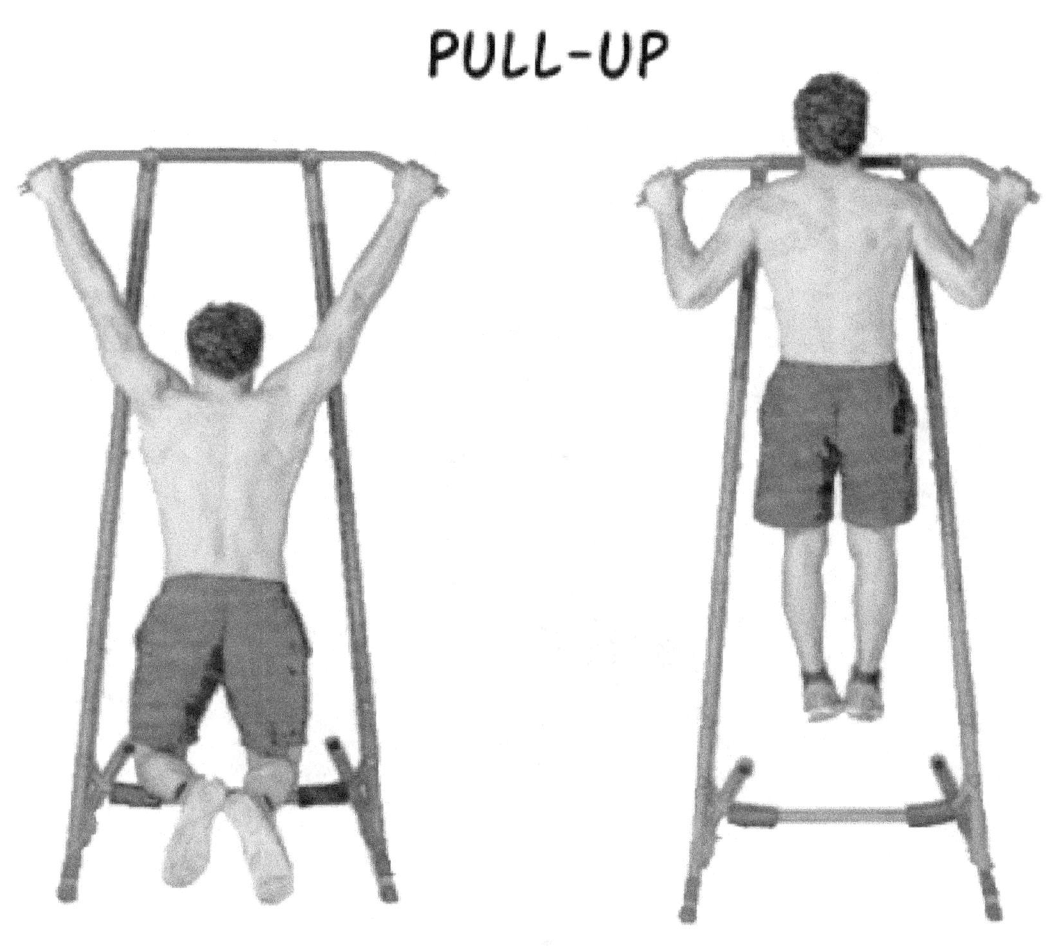

Squats are a great lower-body exercise that works your glutes, quads, and hamstrings. To perform a squat, start by standing with your feet hip-width apart. Bend your knees and lower your body until your thighs are parallel to the ground. Keep your weight in your heels and make sure your knees don't extend past your toes. Return to the starting position and repeat.

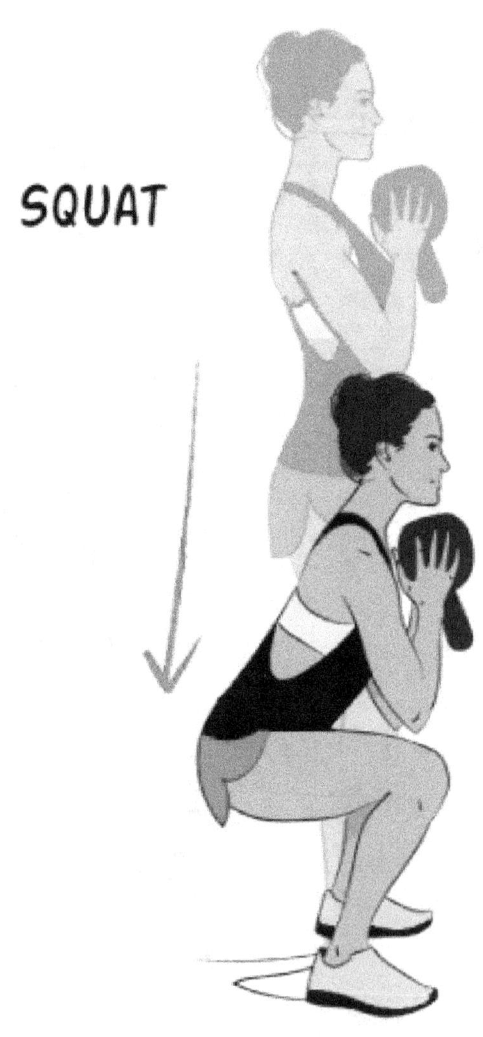

Lunges are an excellent lower-body exercise that works your glutes, quads, and hamstrings. To perform a lunge, start by standing with your feet hip-width apart. Take a step forward with your right foot and bend both knees to a 90-degree angle, keeping your left knee hovering just above the ground. Repeat on the other side.

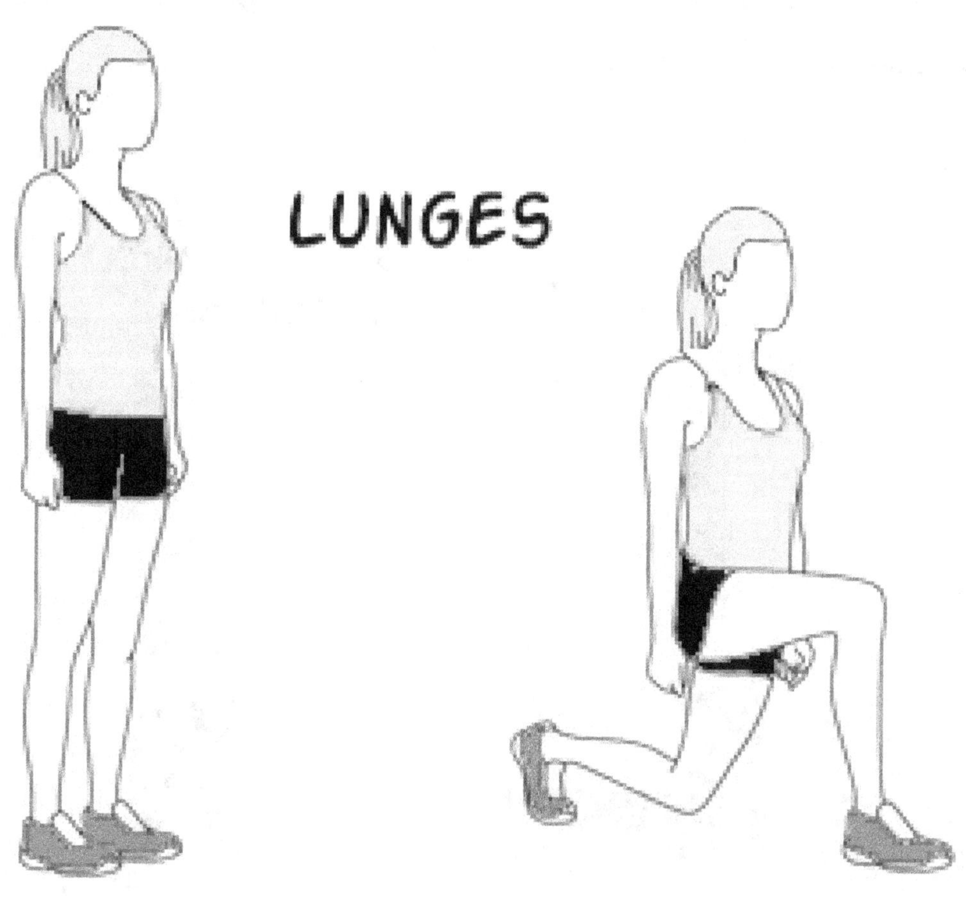

Stomach exercises can help to strengthen the muscles in your abdominal area, which can improve your overall core strength, Reduced risk of injury since strong core can help to stabilize your body during physical activity, reducing the risk of injury to your back, hips, and other areas, Improved appearance strengthening your abdominal muscles can help to tone and firm your stomach area, which can improve your overall appearance and boost your confidence.

There are plenty of stomach exercises but one important point that need to be considered stomach exercise need to be updated regularly.

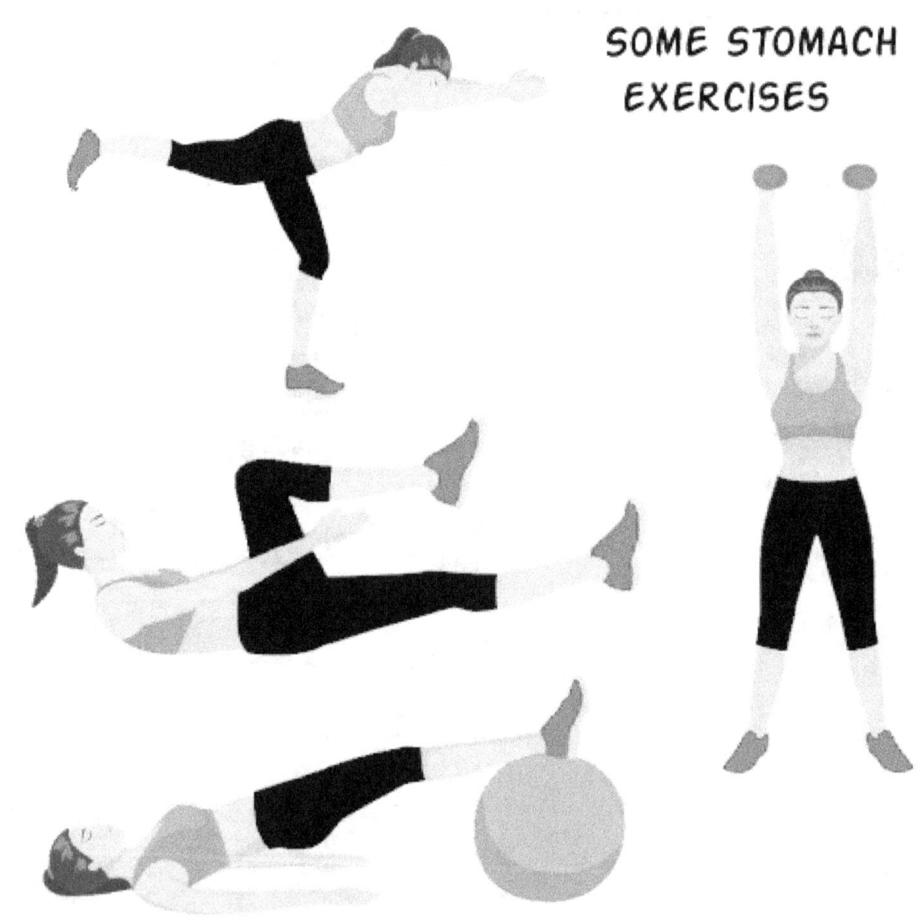

Planks are a fantastic core exercise that can help improve your posture and strengthen your abs, back, and shoulders. Start by getting into a push-up position with your arms straight and your hands shoulder-width apart. Lower yourself down onto your forearms and hold the position for as long as possible. Aim to hold the plank for at least 30 seconds, gradually increasing the time as your strength improves.

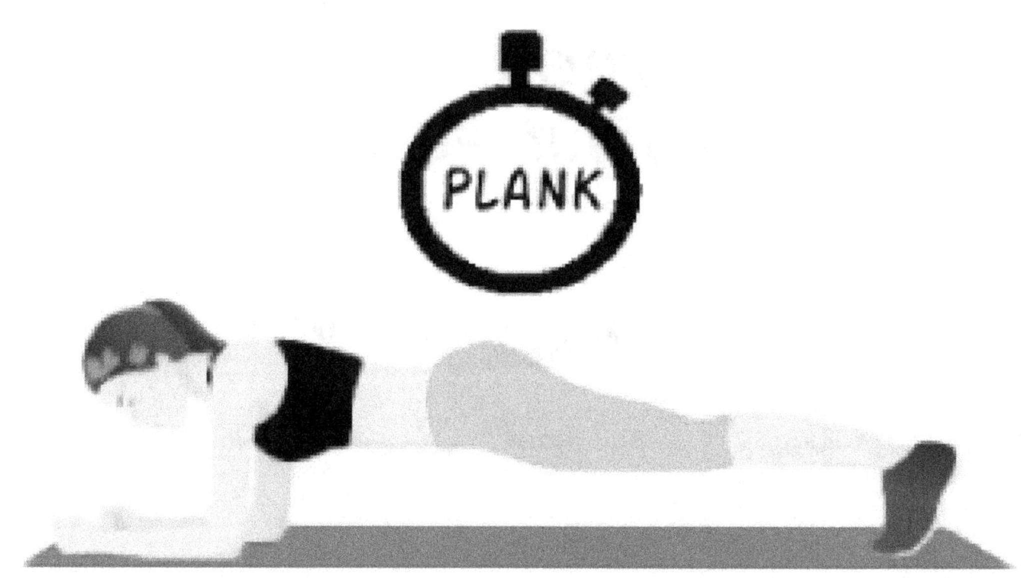

Yoga is an excellent way to improve your flexibility, balance, and overall physical and mental health. There are many different types of yoga, from gentle restorative practices to more challenging vinyasa flows. Some popular poses include downward dog, warrior two, and child's pose.

Note: Yoga needs specialized trainer specially if you are not familiar with, So please take some lessons or hire a trainer or at least watch some videos that can be useful.

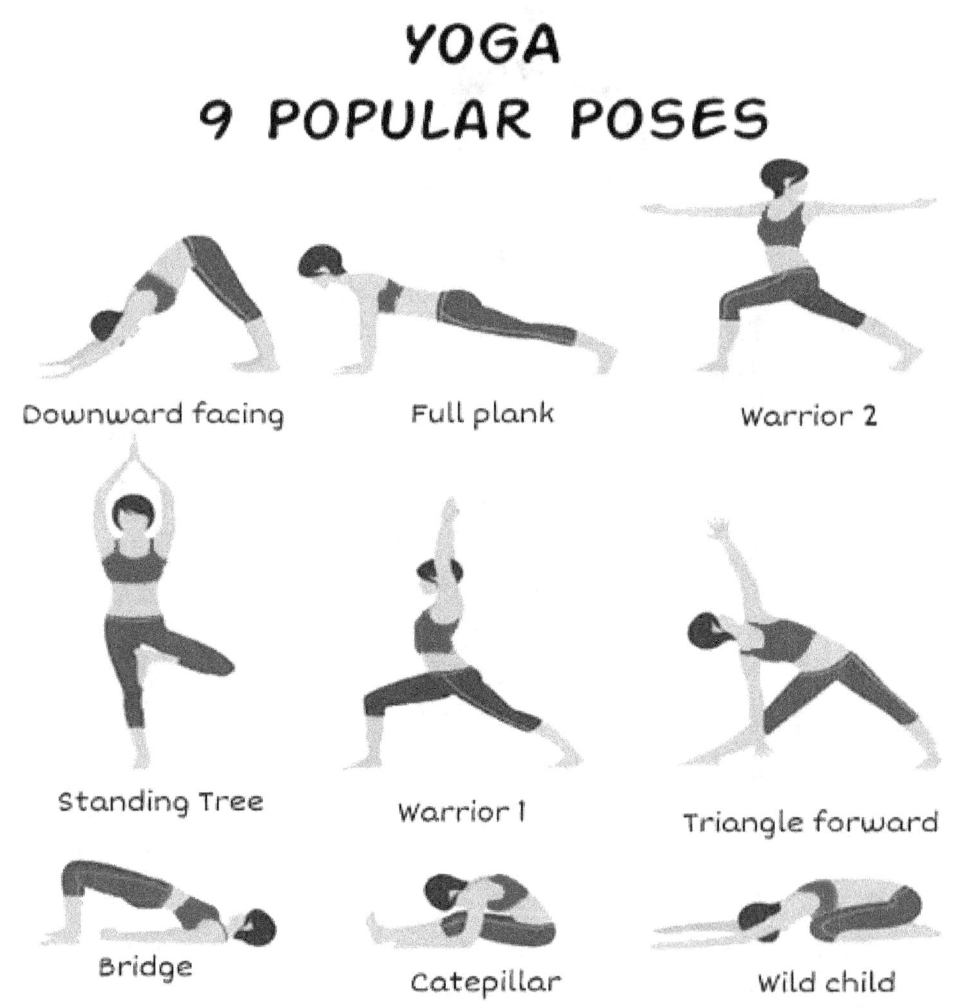

Burpees can help to improve cardiovascular fitness, as they are a high-intensity exercise that can elevate heart rate and stimulate fat burning. Additionally, the exercise can help to build strength, improve coordination and balance, and provide a time-efficient workout that requires no equipment. Burpees can also be modified to suit different fitness levels, making them accessible for people with varying levels of fitness. Overall, incorporating burpees into a regular exercise routine can be a great way to boost fitness and achieve fitness goals.

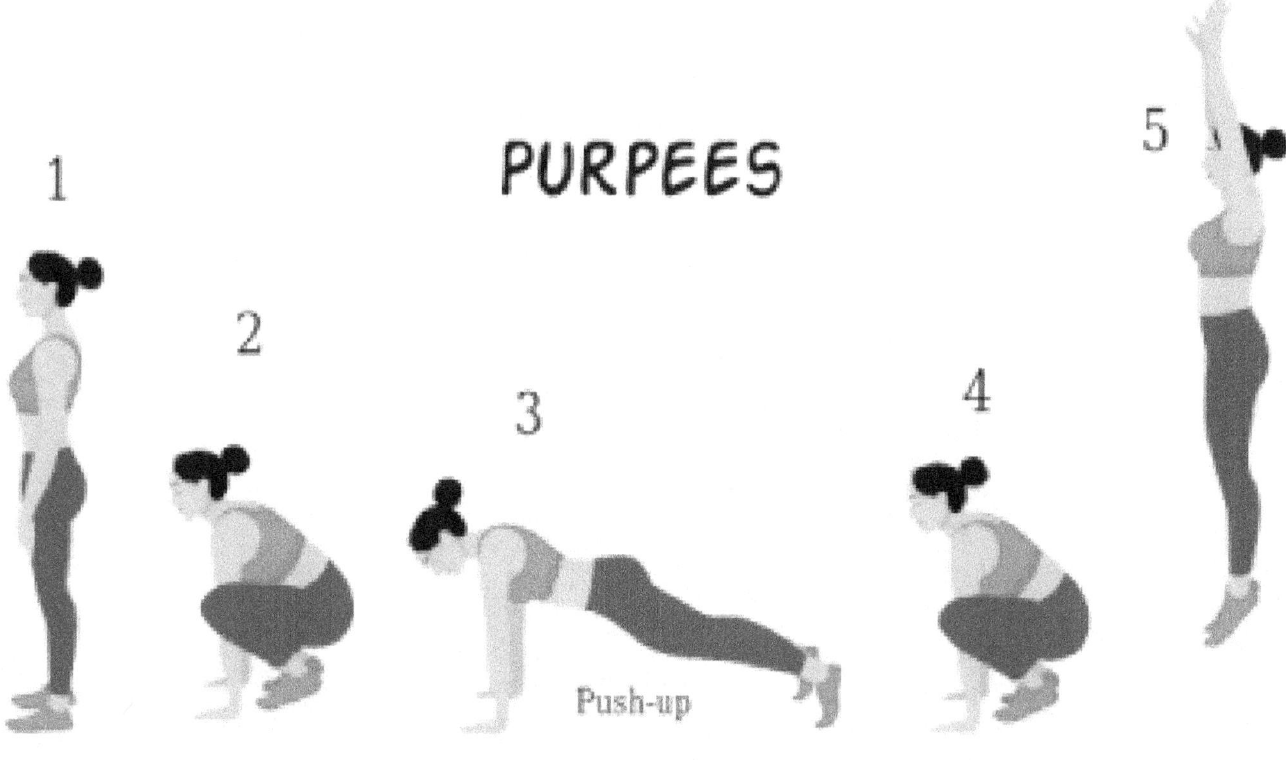

There are many videos and photos out there that can explain all the exercises I have mentioned, it is just easy and popular techniques so it won't be a big challenge to perform these exercises correctly.

Remember, these are just a few examples of the many different types of exercises that can incorporate into morning routines. It's essential to choose exercises that work for your fitness level and personal preferences.

The Science of Morning Exercise

Many studies have shown that morning exercise has significant physical and mental benefits. One of the most significant benefits is the release of endorphins, which are feel-good chemicals that can boost your mood and reduce feelings of anxiety and depression. Endorphins also act as natural painkillers, which can help reduce the discomfort associated with some types of exercise.

Another way that morning exercise can benefit your brain is by increasing blood flow and oxygenation. This can improve cognitive function, memory, and overall brain health. Additionally, regular exercise has been shown to help reduce the risk of age-related cognitive decline and dementia.

In terms of physical benefits, morning exercise can help improve cardiovascular health, increase muscle strength and endurance, and reduce the risk of chronic diseases such as obesity, diabetes, and heart disease. Additionally, regular exercise can help improve sleep quality, which is essential for overall health and well-being.

Overcoming Obstacles

Don't come up with obstacles from nowhere but your own mind, yes that is true.

Starting a morning exercise routine can be challenging, especially if you're not used to waking up early or exercising regularly. However, there are many strategies that you can use to overcome common obstacles and make morning exercise a sustainable habit.

One of the most significant obstacles to morning exercise is fatigue. To combat this, it's essential to establish a consistent sleep routine and aim for at least 7-8 hours of sleep per night. Additionally, you can try gradually shifting your wake-up time earlier over several days or weeks to help your body adjust to the new routine.

Another common obstacle is lack of motivation. To stay motivated, don't put pressure over your back, for example; start jumping rope 20 times then do 5 pushups of three sets, then 3 pull-ups of three sets, then increase gradually every week, three or four months later you will see a huge different, remember that nothing happens at once just one by one also it can be helpful to set specific goals, such as running a 5K or losing a certain amount of weight. Additionally, finding an exercise that you enjoy and look forward to can help keep you motivated and engaged.

Time constraints can also be a challenge, especially if you have a busy schedule. However, by prioritizing exercise and scheduling it into your calendar, you can make it a non-negotiable part of your day. Additionally, choosing shorter, high-intensity workouts can be an efficient way to fit in a workout without sacrificing too much time.

The Importance of Proper Nutrition

Proper nutrition is essential for anyone who wants to get the most out of their morning exercise routine. Eating a balanced breakfast before exercise can help provide the energy and nutrients your body needs to perform at its best. A balanced breakfast should include a mix of carbohydrates, protein, and healthy fats.

Carbohydrates are the body's primary source of energy, so including some complex carbohydrates in your breakfast can help fuel your workout. Examples include whole-grain bread, oatmeal, or fruit.

Protein is essential for muscle repair and growth, so including some protein in your breakfast can help your body recover after exercise. Examples of protein-rich breakfast foods include eggs, yogurt, or protein shakes.

Healthy fats can also provide energy and help keep you feeling full and satisfied. Examples of healthy fats include avocado, nuts, and nut butter.

It's also essential to stay hydrated before, during, and after exercise. Drinking water or a sports drink can help replenish fluids lost during exercise and prevent dehydration.

Anyway, you will see magic change in your breakfast routine if you choose to exercise in the morning, you will notice that you are not into unhealthy food anymore specially on breakfast because you treated your body differently so your body will refuse unhealthy food following the exercise so this was amazing change for me that my body responded to my routine in a healthy way.

The Benefits of Group Exercise

Although I'm exercising by myself but working out with a group or workout buddy can have many benefits, especially for morning exercisers. Group exercise can provide motivation, support, and accountability, making it easier to stick to a regular exercise routine.

Additionally, working out with others can be a fun and social way to exercise. Joining a fitness class or group workout can provide a sense of community and camaraderie, which can be particularly beneficial for those who exercise alone at home to find a morning workout buddy, you can start by reaching out to friends or family members who are interested in fitness. You can also look for local fitness groups or clubs in your area that meet at a convenient time for you.

Another option is to use social media or fitness apps to connect with like-minded individuals who are also interested in morning exercise. Many fitness apps and websites have community features that allow you to connect with others and track your progress together, it's important to find a workout buddy or group that matches your fitness level and goals. This can help ensure that your workouts are challenging but also enjoyable and sustainable.

I have an exercise buddy, she is my wife but she is not as motivated as I am so be careful of negative influencing, even though your exercise buddy decided to stop you have to keep going, it is your health what we talking about here.

Create an Effective Routine That Works for You

Creating an effective morning exercise routine requires planning, consistency, and flexibility. Here are some steps you can take to create a routine that works for you:

Set a specific goal: Identify what you want to achieve through your morning exercise routine. This can help motivate you and provide direction for your workouts.

Choose an exercise that you enjoy: Select an exercise or activity that you enjoy and look forward to. This can help make your workouts more enjoyable and sustainable.

Establish a consistent wake-up time: Try to wake up at the same time each morning to help establish a consistent routine, and this is critical, because if you will be able to stick to a scheduled wake-up time then it will be easier to manage all tasks all over your day.

Schedule exercise into your calendar: Treat your exercise routine like an appointment and schedule it into your calendar to help ensure that it becomes a non-negotiable part of your day.

Start small and gradually increase intensity: Begin with a manageable workout and gradually increase the intensity and duration over time.

Be flexible: Recognize that life happens, and it's okay to adjust your routine as needed. If you miss a morning workout, try to make it up later in the day or the following day, sometimes I cut the training for three weeks due to life pressure but I resumed it back, also I had a surgery once and I had to stop for one and a half month but also, I started all over again.

The Role of Mindfulness and Meditation

Mindfulness and meditation can be powerful tools to enhance the benefits of morning exercise. By incorporating mindfulness techniques into your workout routine, you can improve your mental focus, reduce stress and anxiety, and enhance your overall well-being.

One way to incorporate mindfulness into your morning exercise routine is to practice deep breathing or meditation before or after your workout. Taking a few deep breaths or meditating for a few minutes can help you feel more relaxed and focused during your workout.

Another way to practice mindfulness during exercise is to focus on your body and breath during your workout. Pay attention to your movements, sensations, and breathing patterns, and try to stay present in the moment.

Mindful movement practices, such as yoga or tai chi, can also be beneficial for morning exercisers. These practices combine physical movement with breath awareness and can help improve flexibility, strength, and balance while also promoting relaxation and stress reduction.

How to Stay Motivated

Staying motivated and consistent with your morning exercise routine can be challenging, but there are many strategies you can use to help stay on track.

One key strategy is to set achievable goals and track your progress over time. Celebrate small successes along the way and use them as motivation to keep going.

Another strategy is to find an accountability partner or coach who can provide support and encouragement. This could be a workout buddy, a personal trainer, or an online fitness community.

It's also essential to mix up your workouts and try new exercises or activities to prevent boredom and maintain motivation. Set yourself challenges, such as trying a new workout each week or working towards a specific fitness milestone.

Finally, remember to be kind to yourself and recognize that setbacks and challenges are a natural part of the process. Use these experiences as opportunities to learn and grow, and keep moving forward towards your goals.

Real-Life Examples

The benefits of morning exercise aren't just theoretical - many people have experienced real-life transformations by incorporating regular exercise into their morning routines. Here are a few examples:

Sara is a busy mom of three I have meet her in the bus while commuting she struggled to find time to exercise. However, after committing to a morning exercise routine, she found that she had more energy throughout the day and was able to better manage the demands of parenting. Additionally, she noticed that her mood improved, and she felt less stressed overall.

John was overweight and struggled with low self-esteem, anyway he is my cousin, However, after starting a morning exercise routine, he was able to lose over 50 pounds and gained a new sense of confidence and self-worth. He also found that exercise helped him to manage his anxiety and depression.

Maria is my colleague who struggled with back pain from sitting at a desk all day. However, after incorporating yoga into her morning routine, she noticed a significant improvement in her posture and flexibility. She also found that she was more focused and productive at work, thanks to the mental clarity that comes from regular exercise.

Remember, these are just a few examples of the many different types of exercises that men and women can incorporate into their morning routines. It's essential to choose exercises that work for your fitness level and personal preferences.

Last not least…It's your turn

When the COVID-19 pandemic hit, I lost my job and life came to a standstill. The days felt endless and boring, with no sense of purpose or achievement. It was a tough time, but I knew I had to do something to break the cycle. That's when I started a morning exercise routine. It wasn't easy at first, but I stuck with it and it became a game-changer for me. Even when I eventually got hired again, I couldn't let go of my routine, so you (me) wake up, ride your bicycle for 15 minutes or in the cold weather just jumping the rope then exercising for another 15 minutes maybe more or less and then you take a shower put your clothes on go to work, think about it at 7:30 or 8:00 in the morning you already achieved something so you will go through the day having a mindset full of positivity, achievement, creativity, these little tasks in your daily routine will be very easy after this start because you followed a different approach.

Please note that is not a motivational speak it is just a real experience I have been through and still running.